Dr. Sebi Alkaline Herbal Medicine

50+ Herbal Treatments to Purify Body, Mind and Spirit. Swithc Off The Genetic Codes That Are Slaying Your Immune System

BY

A. J. Bridgeford

© **Copyright 2020 by (A. J. Bridgeford)- All rights reserved.**

This document is geared towards providing exact and reliable information in regards to the topic and issue covered. The publication is sold with the idea that the publisher is not required to render accounting, officially permitted, or otherwise, qualified services. If advice is necessary, legal or professional, a practiced individual in the profession should be ordered.

- From a Declaration of Principles which was accepted and approved equally by a Committee of the American Bar Association and a Committee of Publishers and Associations.

In no way is it legal to reproduce, duplicate, or transmit any part of this document in either electronic means or in printed format. Recording of this publication is strictly prohibited and any storage of this document is not allowed unless with written permission from the publisher. All rights reserved.

The information provided herein is stated to be truthful and consistent, in that any liability, in terms of inattention or otherwise, by any usage or abuse of any policies, processes, or directions contained within is the solitary and utter responsibility of the recipient reader. Under no circumstances will any legal responsibility or blame be held against the publisher for any reparation, damages, or monetary loss due to the information herein, either directly or indirectly.

Respective authors own all copyrights not held by the publisher.

The information herein is offered for informational purposes solely, and is universal as so. The presentation of the information is without contract or any type of guarantee assurance.

The trademarks that are used are without any consent, and the publication of the trademark is without permission or backing by the trademark owner. All trademarks and brands within this book are for clarifying purposes only and are the owned by the owners themselves, not affiliated with this document.

About the author

A. J. Bridgeford

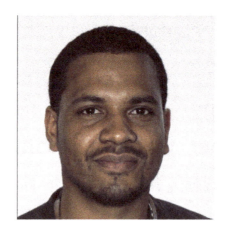

A.J. Bridgeford was born in South Africa and is an incredible traveler who has traveled the globe at least 10 times to discover the wonderful cultures belonging to various countries.

His journey was interrupted when he lost his mother due to an unexpected and terrible illness.

After this happened, he suffered a lot from depression until he realized that his mission was to find a solution to the most well-known diseases and help people in need.

This research led him to Honduras, where he learned and practiced the revolutionary methodologies of the great Dr. Sebi.

Since then, his mission has become to disseminate these incredible treatments and work in the field to improve people's lives.

He is still fighting disease thanks to his private clinics with exceptional results. He wanted to bring back some of his most important knowledge in the field of "alkaline-based medicine" with this book.

With the wish for a healthier life, he reported a quote:

"Life is around us, and we are the fruit of life. Like any fruit, we need the natural elements that the earth makes available to us to become ripe and begin to new life".

Table of contents

About the author 4

Introduction 12

Chapter 1 Introduction to Dr. Sebi herbal medicine 14

1.1 Food in this diet 15

1.2 Advantages of the Dr. Sebi Diet 17

Weight Loss Dr. Sebi Diet 17

Efficient Immune System 18

Reduced Disease Risk 18

Stroke and Hypertension Lower Risk 18

Energy 19

Focus improved 19

Chapter 2 Alkaline foods and benefits 21

2.1 Significance of Alkaline 23

2.2 Alkaline Environment supports 24

2.3 Ayurvedic Perspective 25

Chapter 3 Alkaline herbs & natural ways to solve health problems 31

3.1 Alkaline herbs 31

1. Irish Sea Moss 31

2. Burdock Root 31

3. Soursop Leaves. 32

4. Elderberry 32

5. Black Walnut Hull Powder 32

6. Dandelion Root 33

7. Sarsaparilla Root 33

8. Bladderwrack Powder 33

9. Damiana 34

10. Chamomile Flower 34

3.2 Natural means to solve the health problems 35

Chapter 4 Recipes 50

1. Hot garlic ginger Lemonade 50

2. The Ginger Shot That Will Keep Cold and Flu Away 51

3. Turmeric, ginger, & lemon shots 52

4. Carrot apple ginger(Detox juice) 53

5. Tomato carrot radish (Detox juice) 54

6. Orange carrot pineapples (Detox juice) 54

7. Kale cucumber apple (Detox juice) 55

8. Ginger Lemon Immune Boosting Shots 55

9. Morning Wellness Smoothie 57

10. Pineapple turmeric sauerkraut and gut shots 58

11. Hot and spicy fermented salsa 60

12. How to make probiotic-rich water kefir 62

13. Raw, pickled ginger carrots 63

14. How to make crunchy pickles using my secret ingredient 65

15. Vanilla bean and honey kefir panna cotta 67

16. Lemon verbena kombucha 68

17. Ginger beet sauerkraut 70

18. Fermented zucchini pickles 72

19. Jalapeno cilantro sauerkraut 73

20. Apple spice sauerkraut 76

21. Apple ginger sauerkraut with oranges 79

22. Homemade Kimchi 81

23. Cranberry Cleanser 83

24. Cold Buster Citrus Smoothie 84

25. Apple pie smoothie 85

26. Strawberry Banana Smoothie 85

27. Pineapple Kale Green Smoothie......................87

28. Turmeric and Ginger Tropical Smoothie 88

29. Dark Chocolate Banana Smoothie..................89

30. Blueberry Avocado Mango Smoothie 90

31. Healthy homemade lemonade (naturally sweetened)..91

32. Blackberry Mojito 92

33. Avocado and Herb Salad..................................93

34. Fresh herb salad..95

35. Soft Herb Salad 96

36. All-natural tamarind paste 98

37. Fantastic quinoa bread (Dr. Sebi)..................99

38. Tea Recipe Five Flavored Autumn...............101

39. Veggie fajitas tacos..102

40. Psyllium Apple & Lemon Balm Tea 103

41. Aloe Vera Cherry Juice 104

42. Sugar detox smoothie 105

43. Heart-healthy smoothie 106

44. Immunity-boosting soup 107

45. Nori-burritos 108

46. Lemon-Ginger and Chamomile Tea 110

47. Iron power smoothie 110

48. Dr. Sebi's "stomach soother" smoothie 112

49. Dr. Sebi's "veggie-ful" smoothie 112

50. Detox watercress citrus salad 113

51. Cucumber basil gazpacho 114

52. Dandelion strawberry salad 116

53. Wakame salad 117

54. Super hydrating smoothie 118

Conclusion 120

Introduction

Native Honduran Dr. Sebi (Alfredo Bowman), who considers himself as a natural healer, herbalist, and intracellular therapist initially influenced by a herbalist in Mexico, is the motivation behind the Dr. Sebi diet.

Dr. Sebi's methodology is fascinating and includes concentrating on normal, alkaline, herbs, and plant-based foods while moving away from cell-damaging acidic, artificial foods. By adopting Alfredo Bowman's (Dr. Sebi) method, you will avoid mucus buildup, which can contribute to disease development.

The Honduran-based USHA Healing Village founder is Dr. Sebi that offers to heal and tells people how to follow an alkaline lifestyle.

Medical practitioners also assume that the solution to cure illness by using Dr. Sebi's herbs is unsuccessful since they have been trained to trust in the method of treating patients with medication. This thinking pattern resulted in Alfredo Bowman and his impressive herbal compounds being on the front-page headlines and being submitted to the U.S. Supreme Court in New York, charging Dr. Sebi of creating fraudulent claims without a certificate of practicing medicine and treating people.

Though, many persons have reported that the Dr. Sebi diet has greatly enhanced their wellness with Alfredo Bowman's compounds and that the herbal methods to human treatment have performed better than the conventional approach to medicine. Dr. Sebi's thoughts on dietary compounds & herbal therapy are seen all over YouTube, continuing to educate and inspire safe living also after his passing.

For many, Bowman is an icon and the herbalist since he has found a way to treat life-threatening ailments that have been called incurable. For more than 40 years, he has been a herbalist and claims to cure patients with AIDS, asthma, diabetes, eczema, cancer, epilepsy, heart disease, elevated blood pressure, fibroids, inflammation, multiple sclerosis, lupus, and sickle cells.

Chapter 1 Introduction to Dr. Sebi herbal medicine

The Doctor Sebi Diet is basically a plant-based, vegan diet that limits food and hybrids made by man.

The herbalist Dr. Sebi's diet is all about decreasing acidity in your body's foods and mucus. Dr. Sebi claims that you build an alkaline state in the body, which makes it impossible for disease to survive when you do these things.

Your favorite Dr. mucus relief alkaline diet includes consuming from a customized dietary guide, and food selection focused on 40 + years of study recognizing non-hybrid, alkaline foods while often indulging in a cell food herbal essence.

Naturally, while eating Dr. Sebi's plant-based, alkaline diet, most people lose weight, and they exclude waste, dairy, meat, and refined food from the diet.

In order to assist with cleansing, curing a cell or two, or wellbeing overall, people also mix fasting & herbs with the

Dr. Sebi diet. They normally seek a doctor/health care specialist in these situations.

It is not that challenging to adhere to the long-term Dr. Sebi diet once you can move through the start a few days.

However, the initial days will be tough since you would always crave for sugar.

It does not improve that there are junk food choices everywhere, and most restaurants don't have menu offerings that suit this lifestyle.

1.1 Food in this diet

A vegan diet focused on plants, and a niche variant of an alkaline diet (NIH) is the Dr. Sebi diet. Some even take herbs to nurture the cell, support clean it and cure decades of unhealthy eating when adopting the diet.

"Dr. Sebi believes alkaline foods as " electric foods "for the cell and are raw and live foods for" the nation's healing. "Dr. Sebi typically splits down food into 6 categories:

1. Live

2. Dead

3. Raw

4. Hybrid

5. Narcotics

6. Genetically modified

Herbalist Sebi states that when keeping away from 3 to 6, you can concentrate on numbers 1 and 3 (live and raw). This involves avoiding fruits (seedless), crops weather-resistant like corn and something with additional minerals and vitamins that may be problematic for individuals since there are too many fruits and vegetables sold in grocery stores that are hybrid and GMO genetically modified.

According to Dr. Sebi, non-starchy vegetables, ripe fruit, raw nuts and grains, and butter are foods advised for people who want to live healthily. In the Dr. Sebi diet, leafy greens, rye, quinoa, and Kamut may also play a significant role.

Adverse effects on the human body are caused by acidic foods, like poultry, meat, seafood, or foods involving yeast, sugar, iodized salt, alcohol, or something that is fried.

It can help to cure you of the harmful results acid causes by swapping acidic foods with the electric alternatives.

It can sound unappetizing to acidic humans to follow only raw diets, but when you clean your cells of contaminants, you eventually begin to get accustomed to a raw diet, contributing to the disease cure.

1.2 Advantages of the Dr. Sebi Diet

Reducing acid in food tends to suppress the body's mucus, which develops an alkaline condition that makes it extremely difficult for the diseases to develop. It's much easier to use herbs in the cleansing strategy.

Weight Loss Dr. Sebi Diet

It's self-explanatory. When adopting the diet, weight loss is expected to happen since Dr. Sebi's diet is comprised of natural fruits, vegetables, nuts, grains, and legumes.

It removes waste, meat, dairy, and packaged foods, so you'll lose weight naturally. Dr. Sebi's diet works like a cleanse and reaps several advantages, such as the body thanks you.

Efficient Immune System

The effect of diseases and infections is a poor immune system. Some report that by diligently adopting the Dr. Sebi diet, they've improved their immune system & have been cured of such diseases, and we know that medication doesn't cure illnesses.

Reduced Disease Risk

Acidic foods weaken the mucous layer of the body's cells and inner walls, resulting in a weakened system that renders illness possible and difficult to treat. As a consequence, consuming alkaline diets will decrease the likelihood of illness and help the body get what the healthy cells need to fuel them.

Stroke and Hypertension Lower Risk

The first-line treatments for all levels of hypertension require exercise and weight reduction, according to the NIH. However, the findings of recent cross-sectional analyses show that the most effective intervention than medication and conventional medical practice is a plant-based diet. In contrast to medication, Everyday Health has addressed the advantages of a plant-based diet, noting that a plant-based diet will reduce plaque in blood vessels and lower the risk of diabetes, stroke, and cardiac disease in the medical study they also examined.

As we discussed, a niche variant of a plant-based vegan diet is the alkaline Dr. Sebi diet.

Energy

dairy, meat, and white sugar diets can burden the body and levels of energy. It is a healthier way to concentrate on plant-based eating, which will increase the strength you display on a daily basis.

Focus improved

Following Dr. Sebi's teachings would help clear the brain fog, hold you centered, and be less distracted by stressful conditions that occur.

And if you are not ill, it will help you maintain a long and safe life by using a plant-based approach.

Chapter 2 Alkaline foods and benefits

Getting an alkaline condition in the body allows the various systems that hold pathogens at bay to operate smoothly.

The alkaline Environment, according to Ayurveda, pacifies all doshas.

Satvik food, pranayam, appropriate hydration, accurate meal timings allow the body to retain the acid-alkali balance.

Alkaline foods

Seasonal fruits, fresh salads, citrus, superfoods, mineral water, dairy, and herbal tea are alkaline foods.

Acidic foods

Meat and fish, items that are frozen, packaged, and ready to consume, fried foods create an acidic environment.

Litmus test

A basic home urine/saliva test allows you to decide whether the body is alkaline or acidic.

The basis of longevity and health is an alkaline diet. Today, we are subject to different stressors, rendering our bodies increasingly acidic than ever before, growing stress, contaminated air, and water, food containing additives and preservatives, processed food deprived of natural antioxidants, etc.

The body has a normal mechanism to maintain alkaline, so it tends to leach Ca out of soft tissues to render blood alkaline if the alkaline ions buffer from the body is depleted. Magnesium is further reduced, which contributes to heart disease, joints, muscles, and calf pain. At the origin of nearly all physical disorders is the acid-alkali balance.

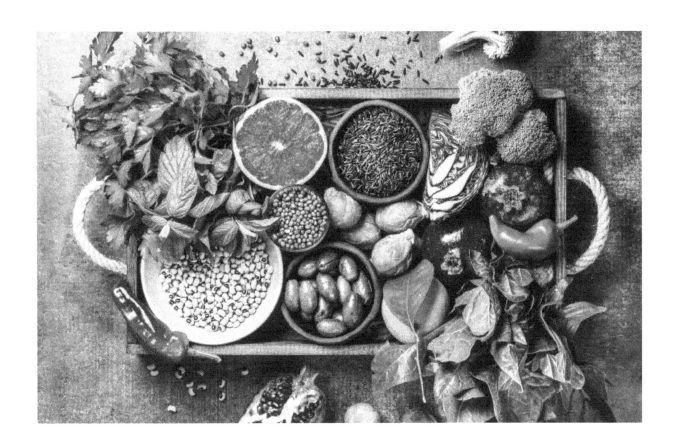

2.1 Significance of Alkaline

- For the correct functioning of body functions, an alkaline body (pH between 7.35 to 7.45) needs to be maintained.

- Essential for strength and defense, for example, the production of cancer cells in an acidic environment.

- Vata & Pitta are aggravated by an acidic diet. All three doshas are pacified by alkaline food.

- All the alkaline foods are easy to digest and provide a cooling or calming impact on the body.

- Alkaline diets contribute to skin that is healthy. The symptoms of the acidic body are premature wrinkles, freckles, lines, and dryness.

2.2 Alkaline Environment supports

- All herbs, most vegetables, and spices are alkaline, while all meats, condiments, intoxicants, canned, and processed foods are quite acidic.

- A diet that comprises of 80% fresh vegetables & juices, legumes, millets, whole grains, seeds, fruits, and nuts 20% can help push the body in an alkaline state from cooked foods and beans.

- Strong alkaline foods such as lime, onion, ginger, apple cider vinegar, garlic, turmeric, virgin coconut oil cold pressed, moringa leaves

- It is also advantageous to consume raw vegetables. Includes vegetable juices as they help build healthy cells in the provision of live enzymes.

- Use fish & lean chicken if you've to, to minimize or prevent meat consumption. Red meats such as pork and beef are cut down because the foods are difficult to digest, and the removal of toxins is slowed down.

- Stop caffeine-loaded beverages such as coffee, black / milk tea, chocolate, etc. Turn back to chamomile, herbal, green tea.

- Reheating the food (for example, in a microwave) will turn the food acidic.

- It is advised to provide the right gap between meals, 3.5 to 4 hrs or at least until the previously consumed meal is already digested. Eating gradually and chewing the food properly helps hold it alkaline.

- At least drink 5-6 water glasses a day for optimal water consumption. With lime & cucumber, or different herbal infusions, water may be turned alkaline.

2.3 Ayurvedic Perspective

Ayurveda's sage physicians did not call pH acidity and alkalinity. They named it Vipaka (the result of the food — the final phases of digestion). Ayurveda strongly emphasizes the intake of alkaline food; according to it, Kshara Vipaka (alkaline effect) or Madhura grants an individual the best health.

- Ayurveda considers all the dairy products (Indian A2 cow) produced from cow's milk to be alkaline.

- Avocados & coconuts are alkaline, as sprouted beans, rock salt, and vegetables such as cucumber, spinach, and broccoli

- Before ingestion, all citrus fruits are acidic, but after and during ingestion, they are alkaline.

- Very alkaline food is Indian gooseberry (Amla or Amlaki). Vata, Kapha, and Pitta are pacified by it. It is bitter, but it leaves a sweet aftertaste, like honey.

Easy tests to decide whether our system is alkaline or acidic

There are a few easy methods to evaluate if the body is alkaline or acidic. These measurements are conducted in the safety of your home using a pH strip.

Testing Your pH Level

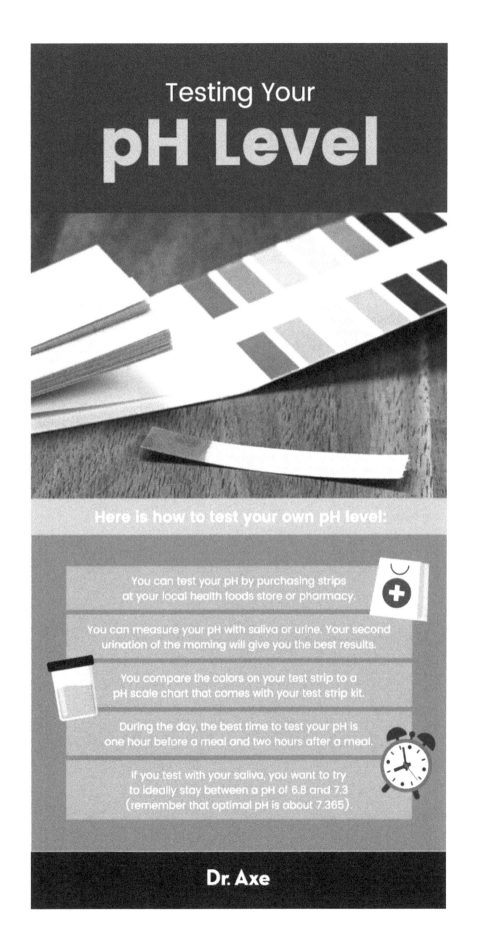

Here is how to test your own pH level:

You can test your pH by purchasing strips at your local health foods store or pharmacy.

You can measure your pH with saliva or urine. Your second urination of the morning will give you the best results.

You compare the colors on your test strip to a pH scale chart that comes with your test strip kit.

During the day, the best time to test your pH is one hour before a meal and two hours after a meal.

If you test with your saliva, you want to try to ideally stay between a pH of 6.8 and 7.3 (remember that optimal pH is about 7.365).

Dr. Axe

pH levels checking

At any drug shop, the pH strips are readily accessible. For verifying if the body is alkaline or acidic in nature, analyses of urine and saliva are done.

Urine examination

Taking the sample of urine early in the morning produces a decent test as you wake up. Dip litmus paper in it and note the shift of color. Compare the change of color to the provided color scale with the litmus paper.

Saliva

Before brushing/consuming or drinking something, gathering the freshly developed saliva in the morning provides a fairly precise test.

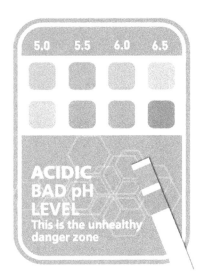 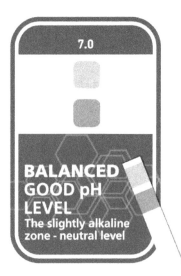 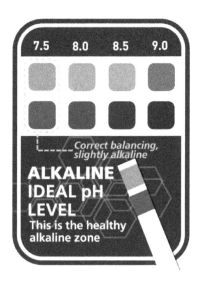

If the diseases can be held away by maintaining an alkaline environment, then the basic lifestyle adjustments offered above can be easily adopted. Preventing diseases rather than curing them makes greater sense. Prevention is far better than treatment

Chapter 3 Alkaline herbs & natural ways to solve health problems

3.1 Alkaline herbs

Herbs, together with a conscientious lifestyle, have power. Here are the best ten Alkaline Herbs

1. Irish Sea Moss

As a facial mask, you can use Irish Sea Moss Gel to your face, which leaves your skin feeling moisturized and smooth. Irish Sea Moss is a perfect source for vitamin supplementation since it includes more than 100 minerals that are important for the human body.

2. Burdock Root

One of the main herbal teas is Burdock Root. This contains all of the body's 102 minerals, but at low levels. We are really much drink this herbal tea as it serves like a "blood cleanser," cleanses your lymphatic system, and functions as a natural laxative as well. There's a really slight earthy flavor to Burdock root that We enjoy.

3. Soursop Leaves.

One of the favorite herbal teas is Soursop Leaves. Soursop is popularly recognized for its anti-cancer & anti-parasitic effects. Soursop leaves go well with ginger, and for a great taste and anti-inflammatory drink, It is normally brewed together.

4. Elderberry

When you've got a cold and just want to give the immunity the boost, elderberries are perfect. Elderberries always help push the immune system but beware of how much as too much you eat might render you nauseous. Elderberries are a perfect addition to brewing tea with other herbs and is also useful for producing cough medicine.

5. Black Walnut Hull Powder

With its antibacterial, antiviral & anti-parasitic effects, it is perfect. This powder is added in the smoothies, or you can turn it in a tea as an option.

6. Dandelion Root

if you really want anything that feels similar to coffee, the dandelion root is great. Put hemp milk & date sugar, and you've got a latte that helps the liver cleanse. Coffee is acidic, but We prescribe it to coffee drinkers every morning as it cleanses the liver, ensuring it gives the energy to you as well (if that's why you drink coffee). A great way to detox and begin the morning is Dandelion Root.

7. Sarsaparilla Root

It is the richest in iron and thus suitable for requiring it. With other spices, like burdock root/dandelion root, Sarsaparilla goes well.

8. Bladderwrack Powder

For thyroid problems, arthritis, artery hardening, stomach diseases, heartburn, blood cleaning, constipation, urinary tract problems, bronchitis, and anxiety, Bladderwrack is used. Genuinely, because of its tremendous minerals and its ability to help strengthen the immune system and improve efficiency, We use Bladderwrack material. Apply smoothies to this powder, and you can barely taste it.

Bladderwrack powder is sometimes used on the skin. Bladderwrack is healthy for the skin and incorporates properties that are anti-aging.

9. Damiana

People like Damiana because when they feel mentally unbalanced or upset, it makes them feel comfortable. As a natural aphrodisiac, Damiana is often widely used. Both males and females can use Damiana. Damiana is also a fantastic herb for the ladies as they encounter their menses.

10. Chamomile Flower

Because of its relaxing and mentally stimulating effects, it is one of the favorite teas. As it deals with anxiety and is really calming, Chamomile is a perfect tea to drink a night. For those battling depression, anxiety, and tension, chamomile is a perfect treatment. Chamomile helped many to immensely relieve the depression and to make their sleep well at night.

Test each of these herbs to see which of them fits well for you. For one individual, what works may not actually work for another. It can be helpful to research and listen to someone about what to try but finding things out about yourself is the perfect way to learn what's right for you.

3.2 Natural means to solve the health problems

Natural treatments for health are getting a significant moment right now on the wellbeing scene. Your store can be a fairly successful spot to locate health remedies, whether it's oil pulling to treat a myriad of problems or using apple cider vinegar to the face to clear up acne.

So, continue reading if you want to find out natural remedies to basic health problems. Right here, we've rounded up Fifty of our picks.

Bad breath: Try the oil pulling.

Try this if you feel like avoiding getting up near with individuals for fear of your bad breath and flossing and brushing twice a day does little to improve. Oil pulling followers swear by the procedure's potential to freshen breath for even longer than a gum or an Altoid. Simply swish the coconut oil around a tbsp for 20 mins per day before brushing your teeth.

Cold & Flu: Dark Leafy Greens

"Jessica Sepel, nutritionist & Instagram sensation, advises consuming dark, leafy greens & Vitamin C to reduce colds or flu:" I'm a true believer in the whole foods in providing immune protection. Dark, leafy greens always are mine go-to.

Vitamin C is a favorite on my desk when to supplements it comes, and it targets the virus's nucleic acid, and it continues hitting the infection until it's gone. Many people use Vitamin C Whole Foods as it's made from beautiful sources of whole food such as Acerola Cherry, Amla Berry, and Camu Camu. They are more bio-available to the bodies, and they are whole foods, which potentially enhances their immune-boosting abilities.

PMS: Try using Magnesium

For many women, Magnesium is crucial in alleviating PMS symptoms. "It helps ease and calm the muscle, which helps the cramps," Sepel says.

For a natural dosage of Magnesium, look at foods, including sunflower seeds, almonds, and vegetables like broccoli and spinach.

Indigestion: Use peppermint

To relieve digestive problems such as indigestion, gas, nausea, and cramps, peppermint, peppermint oil, and peppermint tea are important.

Thin, fragile nails: Consider massaging your nails with coconut oil.

Ditch the chemicals for genuine coconut oil.

Anxiety: Use meditation

If someone suffers from anxiety before they start taking drugs, this will pay off to pursue meditation, here's how. People with an elevated risk of cardiovascular disease, sleep disorders, weight gain, and concentration and memory decline have been related to persistent stress. Regular therapy has also been reported in research to better control the effects of depressive disorders, sleep disturbances, depression, cancer, and cardiac disease. Actually, meditation works, so you can try it.

Dry, flaky skin: seek honey

Not only is it affordable in the beauty line than everything else, but honey also softens & moisturizes dry skin, and it can be directly applied to trouble areas.

Headache: Give acupuncture a shot.

Since the beginnings of Conventional Chinese Medicine, acupuncture is used to alleviate headaches. A 2009 research found that acupuncture helps decrease the severity and frequency of frequent sufferers of headaches.

Weight issues: Pursue healthy fat for weight problems

Sepel advises adding more healthier fats into the diet and eliminating something labeled as low-fat/fat-free if you have been gaining weight gradually, and it won't appear to budge.

Sugar is loaded with reduced-fat and fat-free, and the body absorbs excess sugar as fat. Don't forget about healthier fats such as avocado, nuts, olive oil, and seeds- they provide you a boost of energy and hold you full longer, And they're filled with fiber and vitamin B- that help purify the bloodstream to continue to enjoy vegetables. A healthy body is a lean body, "she added."

Pain during periods: Use Vitamin D

Hot water bottles, stretching, and painkillers are all standard approaches to reduce period pain, however here's something you definitely haven't heard about vitamin D. When they were offered an ultrahigh amount of vitamin D 5 days before their next anticipated cycle, a limited group of people who normally felt extreme menstrual cramps reported substantially reduced pain.

Lower back Sore: Consider Pilates

Strengthening the abdominal muscles will significantly boost lower back pain by muscle-lengthening activities like Pilates.

Eczema: Pursue baths of Magnesium

It is known that magnesium bath salts cure eczema.

Headaches: Use the peppermint oil

For treating a headache, peppermint oil is also added to the skin. Peppermint oil may induce surface warmth as it is added to the skin, which relieves discomfort under the skin.

Stress: avoid caffeine.

Caffeine raises adrenaline inside the body and may trigger discomfort, so if you feel tense, stop it.

Sore muscles: Go for ice therapy

Although a warm bath can provide instant relief to exhausted, overworked muscles, icing with ice wrapped in a wet towel usually avoids more injury to the muscle and will speed up the recovery phase of the muscle.

Joint pain or Arthritis: Consider Turmeric

Turmeric is a yellow herb that has been used for 2,000 years in Ayurvedic medicine in India and China. Anecdotal research suggests that it is beneficial in the treatment of soft tissue inflammation in cases of arthritis. Try turmeric tea, or while cooking, sprinkle it over the food.

Infections of the urinary tract: consider starting liver detox cleanse.

Although the dosage of antibiotics recommended by the doctor can typically remove the urinary tract's inflammation, Sepel states that they may often be a symptom of candida, which could naturally be helped.

To wash away the system, we suggest a liver-detox cleanse. She said that my 'Restart Plan' is an easy, healthy, and really delicious way to cut some of the inflammatory, sugary foods that feed the yeast and relieve frequent UTIs.

Hangover: Consider bananas and coconut water

Coconut water is a strong hydrator that is essential to drinking after a long night out and has 5 electrolytes that our bodies require: potassium, sodium, phosphorus, Magnesium, and calcium. When you consume alcohol, the body still lacks potassium, and bananas will let you replenish it.

Vertigo: Use basil

a common remedy for vertigo aromatherapy is Basil: to the boiling water, add the leaves, and aid with vertigo and breathe in the steam.

Pimples: Use Apple cider vinegar

We enjoy having apple cider vinegar-it works wonders on blemishes. Only rub a bit on the area, and overnight you'll see progress,' Sepel said.

Cravings for Nicotine: Try exercising

Only quit smoking right now. Nice for you. Continue to work out every day for 30 mins — it has been proven to assist with cravings, which might help you quit the habit.

Nausea: Use ginger

For curing nausea and diarrhea, ginger has been used for hundreds of years. For a perfect way to defeat nausea, add some minced, new ginger with lemon in hot water.

Hiccups: Use apple cider vinegar

It has a number of applications, but it has been proven that the strong and sour taste helps get rid of hiccups.

Anemic: Use green vegetables, liver, and red meat.

Low levels of energy. Maybe you would like to check the amounts of iron. It's essential for women to eat lots of iron, so make sure your consumption of leafy green vegetables & red meat is adequately high.

Dry cuticles: use honey, olive oil, and aloe vera

In the cup, mix the raw honey, olive oil, and aloe vera juice, then use as a hand cream and rub the cuticles. Repeat this every week several times.

Infections of the Urinary Tract: Use cranberry juice

Research indicates that the advantageous substances in the cranberry juice could enter the urinary tract to prevent bacterial adhesion inside 8 hours, according to Web MD. However, get to the hospital if recurrent are the UTIs.

Cramps in the muscles: Use Magnesium

Poor amounts of Magnesium contribute to the production of lactic acid, triggering muscle discomfort and tightness. "use both Epsom salt and supplement in baths to get an additional hit of this wonderful mineral as You rest in the shower, "Sepel said.

Body Odor: Consider using chlorophyll liquid

 dark green pigment is Chlorophyll contained in plants that have hemoglobin (the material responsible for carrying oxygen throughout the body) molecular structure. Add a tbsp to your water bottle to improve red blood cells, raise oxygen, increase energy, reduce body odor, protect against cancer, help control bowel motions, increase Magnesium, calcium, folic, and vitamin intake

Asthma: Try vitamin C and fish oil

Many sufferers have learned that increasing their use of fish oil & vitamin C has helped alleviate symptoms.

Sweating: Use potatoes

Nope, we're not offering you a reason to have potato chips. Instead, to stop unnecessary sweating, rub fresh, cut potato under the arms.

Smelly feet: Consider lemon and baking soda.

To control odor, destroy bacteria and fungi and soft the skin, soak the feet in a combination of water, lemon, and baking soda.

Gassy & bloated: Use activated charcoal

It is claimed that activated charcoal is detoxifying and helps to reduce gases.

Pain in the hip: Consider minerals

Osteoarthritis treatment can be assisted by minerals such as boron, copper, silicon, manganese, and zinc.

Cracked heels: On your feet, use hydrogenated vegetable oil.

Clean and dry the feet first and then, as a natural moisturizer, rub the oil onto the heels.

Rosacea: Use anti-inflammatory herbs

An irregular immune or inflammatory reaction is believed to induce rosacea, and some scientific research shows that an anti-inflammatory diet may help reduce the symptoms.

Problems of digestion: Try probiotics and warm lemon water

In the morning, warm water with lemons Sepel suggests: "One of the favorite recommendations is lemons with warm water." Every morning enjoys this hydration raise to ready the body for digestion & detoxification. Probiotics, whether in probiotic-rich foods such as fermented vegetables, organic yogurt, and tempeh or supplement form, are also important. "We still advise to cut gluten for some weeks because for too many, it induces bloating and intestinal pain," she said.

Infected cut: Use honey

It has antibacterial effects and is one of the oldest remedies for cuts and wounds around the world.

Dry, dull hair: Use zinc and silica

For lovely, shiny hair, zinc and silica are essential and are present in so many foods. Silica is important for hair development, "explained Sepel, advising that we" add loads of green leafy vegetables, zucchini, mango, cucumbers, and beans. In items like eggs, pecans, fresh oysters, and Brazilian nuts, zinc is equally essential and can be found. Another must for glossy hair is oily seafood.

Irritable bowel Syndrome: Use peppermint

To relieve IBS, make peppermint tea or eating a peppermint lolly.

Runny nose: Consider rinsing saltwater

In order to get rid of the runny nose, salt and warm water could be what you need.

Insomnia: drink cherry juice

Participants who consumed cherry juice twice in a day fall asleep earlier than the ones consuming a placebo drink in a 2010 study. Give a go-to it

Dandruff: Use baking soda

Swap the baking soda with the shampoo. Just wet your hair, then rub your scalp with baking soda, and rinse. This can reduce dandruff caused by the overly active fungi

Constipation: consume prunes

Thanks to high fiber count and compound named dihydroxy phenyl isatin, which invigorates the intestines & colon into motion, prunes are an age-old home cure when to constipation it comes.

Dry cough: use licorice root tea

Licorice is a conventional cough remedy, although tests have demonstrated contradictory findings as to whether it performs. However, it tastes fantastic, so give it a go

Itchy skin or Rash: Try a mask made of clay

It has been proven that adding to the skin bentonite clay masks helps with itching and a variety of other skin problems, including acne.

Chronic acne: Use processed sugar and dairy out

In order to cope with chronic acne, Sepel recommends ditching milk and refined sugar: "We propose that clients take a 6-week break from the dairy products if they are struggling with chronic acne." Many would find that their redness and inflammation go down pretty fast. Cutting out processed sugar as well,' she added.

Tiredness: use ginseng

Extract of Ginseng is the age-old exhaustion treatment, which you have also found in many energy beverages. Try ginseng tea and dump all the hideous additives in the fizzy energy sodas.

Hair loss: consume more salmon

Salmon, a food that nurtures the hair shaft and cell membranes in the scalp, is a perfect omega-3 fatty acids source. Plus, they strengthen your scalp, which will further avoid your hairbrush from breaking off.

Toenail fungus: Use oil from a tea tree

It is assumed to be successful against many fungi species, and there is plenty of talk on the media world about the ability of the oil.

Chapter 4 Recipes

1. Hot garlic ginger Lemonade

Prep time: 10 minutes Cook time: 30 minutes

Ingredients

- Fresh garlic cloves 3 to 4 - chopped, minced or grated
- Fresh ginger 1 tsp - peel, then mince or grate
- Dried astragalus root 3 pieces - optional
- Cinnamon chips 2 tsp or cinnamon stick 1 small - optional
- Boiling filtered water 4 cups
- Organic lemon 1, juiced
- Honey/organic maple syrup bgrade 2 tbsp

Instructions

1. Garlic & ginger are prepared: peel & chop them.
2. Boil the water in a tea kettle/saucepan.

3. Add minced garlic, astragalus root & grated ginger to a quart-sized mason jar/heatproof glass jar. Place hot water Gently further into mason jar/heatproof glass. Cover it & steep it for around thirty mins.

4. Strain it into different mason jar/glass container using a small hole strainer.

5. To the ginger-garlic combination, Put the one lemon juice and the sweetener of choice.

6. Serve quickly or put in the fridge for later. Serve it warm.

2. The Ginger Shot That Will Keep Cold and Flu Away

Prep. Time: 20 mins

Ingredients:

- Juicy lemons 2 big

- Honey 2-3 tbsp

- Ginger 25 grams – Tools:

Method:

1. Firstly, squeeze the lemon/ lemons to get the juice & strain it. You could even leave its pulp in, but it would also contain small pieces of ginger, so it may be too heavy to drink.

2. Put the honey & lemon juice to the mixer.

3. Roughly cut the ginger and put it to the blender too.

4. For Thirty sec-one min, combine everything. Honey is very dense & we want it to be well blended. Ginger has a rough feel, and it cannot be changed into a paste or anything similar to that quality. You'll even be able to sense a few really tiny pieces of ginger in the shot.

3. Turmeric, ginger, & lemon shots

Prep time 10 mins

Ingredients

- Turmeric root ~7 oz (large handful)

- Lemons 3 to 4, rind removed

- Ginger root ~6 oz roughly chopped

- Sweet apple 1, quartered

- Black pepper (Pinch)

Instructions

1. Mix all the ingredients in a blender then strain out the pulp thru a cloth-lined sieve.

2. To store, place the juice into the bottles, one big jar/ ice cube tray.

3. Put around two ounces into a cup to serve, then put a pinch of black pepper. Now enjoy it.

4. Carrot apple ginger(Detox juice)

Prep time 5 min

Ingredients

- Carrots 2

- Apples 2

- Ginger 2 tbsp

Instructions

1. Mix all the ingredients and blend.

5. Tomato carrot radish (Detox juice)

Prep time 5 min

Ingredients

- Carrots 2
- cherry tomatoes 15
- radishes 2

Instructions

1. Mix all the ingredients and blend.

6. Orange carrot pineapples (Detox juice)

Prep time 5 min

Ingredients

- Orange 1
- carrots 2
- pineapple 1& ½

Instructions

1. Mix all the ingredients and blend.

7. Kale cucumber apple (Detox juice)

Prep time 5 min

Ingredients

- Kale stalks 6
- Cucumber 2
- Apple 1

Instructions

1. Mix all the ingredients and blend.

8. Ginger Lemon Immune Boosting Shots

Prep Time: 7 minutes

Ingredients

- Ginger root 450 gr
- Lemons 6

- Honey 1 tsp or agave/maple

- Cayenne pepper 1/8 tsp

Instructions

1. Begin by scrubbing & cleaning the ginger root. It has to be peeled and cut into a tiny enough section to get through the juicer.

2. Start by juicing the ginger then.

3. If the ginger is juiced, verify the sum of yield as well as the lemons are juiced properly. If you remove the skin & white rind, it may pass it through the juicer. Alternatively, as usual, juice the lemon and weigh a ratio of 1:1 with ginger juice.

4. Mix the juice of lemon & ginger together.

5. Add the honey & the cayenne pepper/agave/ maple, then whisk well to mix it completely.

6. Divide into portions of 60 ml (shot-sized) & refrigerate them for up to one week. The pepper of cayenne will fall

to the floor-so before drinking, be sure to shake the shot bottle.

7. You could even chill the juice into the ice cubes &, if necessary, put it to the smoothies & juices.

9. Morning Wellness Smoothie

Prep Time10 mins

Ingredients

- Small Beets 2, peeled

- Carrots2

- Ginger2 " peeled

- Blueberries1 cup (fresh or frozen)

- Mango2 cups

- Pitted Dates2-3

- Almond Milk1 1/2 cup

Instructions

1. In a mixer, Put all the ingredients, & pulse till mixed. Serve right away.

2. If it is too thick for the smoothie, add more sugar. Add more frozen fruit/ice when it is too thin.

10. Pineapple turmeric sauerkraut and gut shots

Ingredients

- Cabbage head 1 (shredded)
- Pineapple ½ (chopped)
- Ground turmeric 1 tbsp
- Fresh ginger 1 tbsp (grated)
- Sea salt1 tbsp
- Brine
- Sea salt 1 tbsp
- Raw apple cider vinegar1 tbsp
- Purified water 4 cups

Instructions

1. Cut the cabbage with a fine knife in a mixing bowl, mandolin/chop. Put it in a large bowl.

2. Cut the pineapple into tiny bits and then use the cabbage to put it in the bowl.

3. To the bowl, put the minced ginger & sea salt.

4. Massage cabbage combination with the hands for five min or before it begins to break down & becomes tender.

5. Let it sit in the bowl for fifteen min.

6. The cabbage would become very soft & moist within fifteen min. Now, when you squeeze it, there will be juice coming out.

7. Place the curcumin to cabbage. You should either use the hands/spoon to mix it. The curcumin can stain orange on your hands and fingernails so that you might use a spoon.

8. We will make the brine now & put it to the jars for gut shots.

9. Combine one cup of hot water with salt to create the brine. Put the excess water & the apple cider vinegar when the salt dissolves.

10. Onto the mason jars, add the brine, leaving around an inch from its top.

11. In the pot, mix together the cabbage & brine till it's all mixed.

12. Put a cover lightly on the jar so that gas can escape as fermentation occurs.

13. In a cool, shaded spot, put on the counter for 4 to 7 days.

14. The sauerkraut will bubble up somewhat during fermentation & become cloudy. Take it with a spoon if scum emerges.

15. Shake up the mason jar a day or two so that the cabbage dips under the brine & will not grow mold.

16. Put in the fridge & serve cold.

11. Hot and spicy fermented salsa

Prep time 20 mins

Ingredients

- Chopped tomatoes 4 cups
- Jalapeño Peppers 2
- Habanero Pepper 1
- Red Onion ¼, finely chopped
- Garlic Cloves 3
- Pickle Juice ¼ Cup
- Sea Salt 1 tbsp

Instructions

1. Cut the jalapeno peppers, tomatoes, red onion & habanero then place them in a large bowl.

2. Chop the garlic or add it to the bowl by pressing it thru a garlic press.

3. Put sea salt

4. Mix it & put it in a mixer.

5. Add the juice of the pickle.

6. Pulse the combination sometimes till it is smoother & equally chopped up.

7. Place it into a quart diameter mason jar & loosely seal to make it easier for gas to escape.

8. Set out in a cool position away from direct sunshine on the counter for three days.

9. Chill before eating & safe in the refrigerator.

12. How to make probiotic-rich water kefir

Prep time 10 mins

Ingredients

- Water Kefir Grains ¼ Cup
- Brown Sugar ¼ Cup
- Liquid Minerals ½ cap (optional)
- Quart Water

Instructions

1. Halfway mostly with spring water, full the mason jar, put the minerals & brown sugar, then whisk till the sugar dissolves.

2. Put the grains of kefir & finish off with the water left. For 2 days, screw on the lid and sit on the counter.

3. Strain the water kefir into a mason jars/pitcher with a wooden strainer/plastic & put it in the refrigerator. To make more batch, repeat this recipe.

4. Simply drink it or add your preferred juice.

13. Raw, pickled ginger carrots

Prep time 15 min

Ingredients

- Mason jars 2-quart size

- Organic carrots grated5 lb bag

- High-quality sea salt2 tbsp

- Grated ginger6 tsp

Instructions

1. In a mixing bowl or through the hand, mince the carrots. Put them in a large bowl.

2. Add the minced ginger & sea salt.

3. Massage the ginger & sea salt into the carrots for around five min with the hands. Make careful to spread the salt and ginger equally.

4. Let wait for ten min. The salt extracts of the liquid as from carrots, making these moist & limp.

5. Put the carrots strongly with the hands it into a mason jar. Under the liquid, the carrots must be dissolved. When they are an inch from its top of the pot, keep packing throughout the carrots. To hold them underwater under the brine, you could put a weight on top or force them back lower under the brine day-to-day. Cover lightly with a lid so that fermentation gases could escape

6. Let them sit on the counter for 4 to 7 days in a dark spot. Verify that they are not in direct sunshine.

7. If there is a fungus/scrum shows on the top of the carrots, just wipe it off. This is normal & the carrots are still fine under the brine.

8. After four days, taste them. Then place them in the refrigerator if they are tangy & you like the flavor. They'll be comfortably kept for many weeks in the refrigerator.

14. How to make crunchy pickles using my secret ingredient

Prep time 15 mins

Ingredients

- Mason jars 2
- Persian cucumbers about 10 small
- Garlic roughly 1 tablespoon chopped
- Whole peppercorns 1 tablespoon
- Bay leaves 4
- Fresh dill head fronds 2
- Loose-leaf black tea leaves 2 teaspoons

- Brine: sea salt 2 tablespoons, water 4 cups, Bragg apple cider vinegar 1 tablespoon

Instructions

1. Split the ingredients b/w the 2 ball jars, Put the cucumbers to jars & put in the peppercorns, fresh dill, garlic, tea leaves & bay leaves.

2. Create & place the brine into the ball jars, fully surrounding the pickles.

3. By using a neat rock, check the cucumber's weight, a little ramekin, or some such item you may find in the home. To keep them down, use a plastic cover & after that, place a glass ramekin over the highest point of it. For them to remain under the brine is very important, or they may become mold.

4. Seal to hold bugs out with a cover/lid with fabric.

5. See the cucumber after four to five days to check if it's prepared.

6. The pickles are prepared until the brine becomes cloudy; they smell like pickle heaven, & the cucumbers color changes to olive green/yellow.

15. Vanilla bean and honey kefir panna cotta

Prep time 15 mins

Ingredients

- Plain milk kefir 2 cups

- Vanilla bean powder 1 tsp

- Honey 1 tbsp

- Great lakes gelatin powder 2½ tsp

- Hot water ¼ cup of

- Chopped strawberries 3 cups

Instructions

1. Put the kefir & mix the honey & vanilla in a saucepan.

2. Lower the heat & nicely heat up the kefir. You just have to warm it. There will be a risk of destroying the beneficial bacteria if any hotter.

3. Stirring constantly the vanilla & honey once well combined.

4. In a bowl, add the powder of gelatin & place the warm water on it. Mix it till it's dissolved.

5. Smoothly place the gelatin combination into the hot kefir while stirring the kefir.

6. Mix the combination together till it's become creamy & smooth.

7. For some hours or for overnight, place into glasses & cool in the refrigerator.

8. Finely chop the raspberries & put them on the highest point of Panna Cotta then serve.

16. Lemon verbena kombucha

Prep time 20 mins

Ingredients

- Green tea kombucha ½ gallon(

- Fresh lemon verbena leaves 2 cups

- Hot water 1 cup

- Sugar 1 tablespoon

Instructions

1. Carry one glass of water to simmer.

2. For fifteen min, boil the lemon bee brush leaves in warm water.

3. Strain out the leaves and put some sugar. Mix till dissolved.

4. Allow the warm tea to cool at room temp.

5. To a broad pitcher, put the chilled lemon verbena tea & simple kombucha then mix.

6. Fill up the flip-top bottles with the kombucha by using a funnel.

7. Wrap the bottles then let them sit for three to seven days in a dark & cool place.

8. Verify 1 of the bottles after three days & if it's bubbly, place it in the refrigerator. Only serve cold

9. Keep it out for a couple more days if it is not bubbly. Till it is carbonated, review every day.

10. Safe it in the refrigerator & serve it cold.

17. Ginger beet sauerkraut

Prep time 15 mins

Ingredients

- Beets grated 3

- Cabbage head 1 shredded

- Ginger peeled 1" and thinly sliced/grated

- Sea salt 1 tbsp

Instructions

1. Take three outer leaves from the cabbage head. In a mixing bowl/mandolin, chop leftover cabbage. Mince the ginger & beets, then place it in a large bowl & add salt.

2. Massage the cabbage combination by using the hands till it collapses & becomes tender (approximately five minutes). After that, allow it to rest for ten mins to give it time to collapse further and produce further juices.

3. Cover the cabbage firmly in the mason jar, pressing it the whole way down till it falls into its own juices. Leave the space about 11/2 inches from the highest point of the jar. Add additional brine by mixing a tsp of sea salt with one 1 glass of water if there is insufficient brine to fill the cabbage.

4. To move the cabbage under its brine, roll leaves up and put them within a jar. Screw lightly on the jar so that gas could escape when fermentation happens. In a shaded cool spot, put on a counter for five to seven days. The sauerkraut would bubble up somewhat during fermentation & turn cloudy. Remove it with the spoon if scum emerges.

5. Remove the cabbage leaves that are folded up & toss before serving.

18. Fermented zucchini pickles

Prep time 20 mins

Ingredients

- Zucchini 4 cups thinly sliced in rounds
- Med sized red onion ¼ thinly sliced
- Garlic gloves smashed 3
- Grated ginger 2 teaspoons
- Filtered water 4 cups
- Fine Celtic sea salt 2 tbsp or other sea salts of high quality
- Ground turmeric ½ tsp
- Half gallon jar 1 or quart-sized jars 2

Instructions

1. Cut the Courgette thinly into circles.
2. In a half mason jar, put the Courgette rounds or divide b/w smaller jars.

3. Add the garlic, ginger & red onion.

4. Adding half a cup of hot water with the salt makes the saltwater brine & whisk till the salt fully dissolved.

5. When the salt is dissolved, put the leftover water to the saltwater. Place the turmeric & stir well.

6. Place the Courgette & the brine within the jar. There should be plenty for the Courgette to be submerged below the brine.

7. Close the jar lightly with a cover & keep it for three to seven days in a dark, dry position away from the intense sunlight.

8. Check the Courgette to see if it's prepared when the brine is ready. It's meant to be salty, and it smells like pickles.

9. You can store it in the fridge for a month.

19. Jalapeno cilantro sauerkraut

Prep time 30 mins

Ingredients

- Cabbage head 1 shredded

- Sea salt 1 tablespoon

- Jalapeños 4, seeds removed

- Garlic cloves 2

- Cilantro ½ cup

- Onion ½

- Mason jar Quart size/fermentation crock

Instructions

1. Drag three outer leaves it off the cabbage head & set them aside. Chop the leftover cabbage with a knife in a mixing bowl/mandolin. Put it in the large bowl.

2. For around five min, season the cabbage with salt & combine then massage the salt further into the cabbage.

3. Put aside the cabbage and let it rest for fifteen to twenty mins because there is time for the sea salt to drain the liquid out & to turn the cabbage tender.

4. After that, at a med flame, extract the seeds from jalapenos or rather leave them for the spicier kraut & put them in a mixing bowl. Be cautious while handling the peppers, as the skin and eyes could burn & irritate them. While handling this, you should wear gloves & wash your hands quickly afterward.

5. Put the cilantro, onion & garlic to the mixing bowl also and combine till all the ingredients are thinly minced.

6. Move back to cabbage & use your hands to combine & squeeze the cabbage once more. It is prepared for another move if liquid falls out when pressed.

7. Put the cabbage to the jalapeño combination & stir it all up. Use the hands unless you're wearing gloves; use the spoon otherwise.

8. Place your cabbage in the ball jar firmly with a vegetable pounder/gloved hand. Force this all the way back down till it submerges with its own fluids.

9. Do this till there is a space of about 1 1/2 inches from the jar's highest point.

10. To force the cabbage under the brine, fold up the leaves & put them in the jar.

11. Screw lightly on the jar so that gas could escape when fermentation happens. In a shaded & cool spot, put on the counter for five to seven days. In the case that it spills over and creates a mess, put a plate under the ball/mason jar.

12. The sauerkraut would bubble up somewhat during fermentation & turn cloudy. Clean it with the spoon if scum emerges.

13. Remove the cabbage leaves that are folded up & toss before serving.

14. Place it in the refrigerator.

20. Apple spice sauerkraut

Prep time 30 mins

Ingredients

- Cabbage head 1

- Fine Celtic sea salt 2 tablespoons/other salts of high quality

- Apples shredded 3 medium (about 3 cups)

- Fresh grated ginger 1 tablespoon

- Ground cinnamon 1 tsp

- Ground cloves ¼ tsp

- Mason jar quart size 1 or 2 small glass jars

Instructions

1. Drag three outer leaves it off the cabbage head & set them aside. Chop the leftover cabbage with a knife in a mixing bowl/mandolin. Put it to the large bowl.

2. For around five min, season the cabbage with salt & combine then massage the salt further into the cabbage.

3. Put aside the cabbage and let it rest for fifteen to twenty mins because there is time for the sea salt to drain the liquid out & to turn the cabbage tender.

4. Chop the apples by using the food processor/mixing bowl.

5. To the cabbage combination, Put the ginger, chopped apples, cloves & cinnamon.

6. Using the hands/vegetable pounder to combine & push the cabbage combination until the liquid falls out when pressed.

7. Firmly place the cabbage in the ball/mason jar. Force this all the way back down until it submerges with its own fluids using vegetable pounder or the hands.

8. Do this till there is a space of about 1 1/2 inches from the highest point of the jar.

9. To force the cabbage under the brine, fold up the leaves & put them in the jar.

10. Screw lightly on the jar so that gas could escape when fermentation happens. In a shaded & cool spot, put on the counter for five to seven days. In the case that it spills over and creates a mess, put a plate under the ball/mason jar.

11. The sauerkraut would bubble up somewhat during fermentation & turn cloudy. Clean it with the spoon if scum emerges.

12. Remove the cabbage leaves that are folded up & toss before serving.

13. Safe it in the refrigerator.

21. Apple ginger sauerkraut with oranges

Prep time 25 mins

Ingredients

- Purple cabbage head 1 shredded

- Green apples 2 chopped in thin slices

- Orange 1 sliced in rounds

- Ginger grated 2" or ginger juice ¼ cup.

- Sea salt 1 tablespoon

- Pure water

Instructions

1. Peel off the cabbage's 2 outer leaves & put them aside. In a large bowl, put the leftover cabbage, ginger, sea salt & apples.

2. Stir & rub the cabbage combination for around five min with the hands. The cabbage is going to start breaking down and getting muddy. That's the brine here. In a big glass container/mason jar, pack the cabbage combination.

3. Continue to put the combination of cabbage & oranges until the surface has around 2-3 inches of space, & after that, fill the jar with distilled water till the cabbage is just covered.

4. Fold up the cabbage leaves & put them on the combination's top. This is used just under the water line to carry the sauerkraut. Cover it & put it for five to seven days in a dry & cool place.

5. To allow the gas out produced by the fermentation, open the cover everyone to two days.

6. After five to seven days, place it in the refrigerator, and enjoy your meals.

22. Homemade Kimchi

Prep time 1.5 hours

Ingredients

- Napa cabbage 1 pound
- Pink salt 3 tbsp
- Water 1-2 cups
- Daikon radish 1/2 cup (julienned)
- Carrot 1 (julienned)
- Green onion 3 stalks

Paste

- Chili flakes 1-3 tbsp
- Fish sauce 1 tbsp
- Sesame oil 1 tbsp
- Cloves garlic 2 (grated)
- Ginger 1/2 "cube (grated)

- Sugar 1 tbsp

Instructions

1. To make more bite-sized pieces, begin by slicing the napa cabbage in fourths widthwise. The cabbage is going to shrink, so don't end up making it too tiny. Leave out the harsh cores & save for a broth later on or discard.

2. Mix the cut cabbage & salt in a big bowl then rub with your hands for around ten minutes. You can see the cabbage starting to wilt & shrink. After this, cover the water only with cabbage & allow it to rest for one hr. To hold it submerged, put a plate with anything strong on top.

3. Mix all the ingredients paste to get the chili paste & combine well to mix. If you want it spicier, put 1 tbsp of chili flakes or three. You may keep the sugar out because when the bacteria feed on sugar, it also helps speed up the fermentation phase.

4. Rinse it below cool water for around five min after the cabbage is finished soaking, ensuring all the leaves are

rinsed. Then put the radish, carrots, the chili paste, + green onion & rub really well onto the cabbage leaves. Hold your gloves on, or your hands are going to burn & discolor.

5. Using very warm water, clean the cover & the jar quite well. Dry them & get ready to fill. Stuff the kimchi as securely as you can into the jar. Be sure to force the contents down to the top of the jar till you see the water simmering.

6. Leave it to ferment for two to five days at room temperature. Sometimes, with a washed spoon, you can reach into the jar & force the contents downward if they appear very dry on top. Put the leftovers in the fridge after eating it.

23. Cranberry Cleanser

Prep time 5 min

Ingredients

- Pear 1

- Apple 1

- Cucumber 1

- Celery stalk 1 Lg

- Handful spinach 1

- Cranberry ½ cup

Instruction

1. Mix in a juicer/blender. This juice functions by washing and removing body fat from the lymphatic system.

24. Cold Buster Citrus Smoothie

Prep Time: 5 minutes

Ingredients

- Peeled oranges 2

- Frozen mango chunks 1/2 cup

- Banana 1

- Coconut water 1/2 to 1 cup

Instructions

1. Use a high-powered blender to mix all ingredients & blitz till blended.

2. Put less/more water of coconut to the consistency required. Enjoy.

25. Apple pie smoothie

Prep time 5 mins

Ingredients:

- Vanilla yogurt 6 oz

- Apple chopped 1

- Milk 1/2 cup

- Honey 1 Tbsp

- Ice cubes 1/2 cup

- Cinnamon 1/4 tsp

Directions

1. In a blender, put all ingredients & blend till smooth.

26. Strawberry Banana Smoothie

These red berries are delicious and are rich in vitamins, fiber, and antioxidants.

Ingredients

- Frozen strawberries 1 cup
- Banana 1/2
- Sliced raw nuts 2 tbsp (almonds, cashews, walnuts, and pecans are excellent sources of fiber, protein, and healthy fatty acids)
- Chia seeds 1 teaspoon
- Granola 1/4 cup
- Unsweetened Greek yogurt 1 cup
- Soy/almond milk /other non-dairy milk 1 cup
- Honey 1 tsp (optional)

Directions

1. In a blender, add all the ingredients & mix till smooth.
2. Place it into cups & serve.

27. Pineapple Kale Green Smoothie

Prep time 5 mins

Like many fruits and veggies, this leafy green contains phytochemicals, which are compounds that protect cells from a range of damages that may lead to health issues like cancer.

Ingredients

- Raw kale leaves 2 cups, stems removed

- Almonds 3/4 cup

- Frozen/fresh banana 1 cup

- Plain Greek yogurt 1/4 cup

- Pineapple pieces 1/4 cup

- Nut butter 2 tbsp (unsweetened)

- Almond milk 1 cup

- Honey 1-2 tsp

Instructions

1. Put all the ingredients into the mixer.

2. Mix all the ingredients till smooth. To make your desired quality, adjust the liquid.

28. Turmeric and Ginger Tropical Smoothie

Prep time 5 mins

This drink is a rejuvenating snack, perfect for a healthy weight loss meal plan. Plus, both ginger and turmeric contain antioxidants and may decrease inflammation markers in the body.

Ingredients

- Almond or soy milk 1 cup

- Fresh/frozen banana ½

- Frozen/fresh mango chunks ½ cup

- Each ½ Tsp. Ground turmeric, cinnamon, ginger, and cardamom

- Flaxseed 1 tsp

- Honey 1 tsp (optional)

- Ice cubes 1/2 cup (optional)

Instructions

1. Put all the ingredients to the mixer.

2. Mix all the ingredients till smooth. To make your desired quality, adjust the liquid.

29. Dark Chocolate Banana Smoothie

Prep time 5 mins

Ingredients

- Frozen banana 1

- Raw spinach 1 cup

- Unsweetened almond milk 1 cup (or milk of choosing)

- Chia seeds 3 tbsp.

- Unsweetened cocoa powder 2 tbsp.

- Vanilla extract 1/2 tsp.

- Honey 1 tbsp. (optional)

Instructions

1. Put all the ingredients to the mixer.

2. Mix all the ingredients till smooth

30. Blueberry Avocado Mango Smoothie

Prep Time 5 mins

Ingredients

- Blueberries 1 cup

- Frozen mango 1 1/2 cups

- Avocado ½

- Chia seeds 1 tbsp

- Matcha powder 1 tsp (optional)

- Unsweetened almond butter, sunflower butter, or cashew butter 2 tbsp

- Coconut water 1½ to 2 cups

- Raw honey 1 tbsp (optional)

Instructions

1. Add all the ingredients to the mixer.

2. Mix all the ingredients till smooth. To make your desired quality, add additional liquid.

3. For a smoothie filling, put 1 Tablespoon of coconut flake granola as a topping.

31. Healthy homemade lemonade (naturally sweetened)

Prep Time: 10 minutes

Ingredients

- Water 6 cups

- 1/3–1/2 cup light-tasting honey or agave

- Fresh lemon juice 1 cup

- Fruit puree Optional

- Few sprigs of fresh mint/basil Optional

Instructions

1. In the saucepan/microwave, heat one glass of water till really hot to touch (but not simmering).

2. Put honey & mix to dissolve.

3. Place the honey combination into the pitcher.

4. Add water & juice of the lemon.

5. Put puree & herbs together with water when using fruit puree/herbs.

6. Mix to combine & taste, adding fresh herbs, more puree of fruit agave/honey as desired.

7. Put the lemonade in the fridge for around one week.

32. Blackberry Mojito

Prep time 5 min

Ingredients

- Fresh blackberries 5 – 6

- Fresh mint leaves 4

- simple syrup/blackberry syrup1 1/2 ounces

- Fresh lime juice 3/4 ounce

- Club soda 1/4 cup, chilled

- White rum 1 to 1 1/2 ounces

- Ice cubes 1 cup

- Garnish with fresh whole blackberries and mint

Instructions

1. In a shallow bowl, add the mint leaves, blackberries, lime juice & simple/ blackberry syrup. Through a muddler, nicely mash your combination. Do not tear the mint leaves, only bruise them so that the essential oils are released. Stir in the soda & rum from the club. Strain to extract the seed of blackberry & mint leaves remnants. Place it into cooled stemware. Sprinkle with a few whole, fresh blackberries & fresh mint sprigs & add ice. Serve.

33. Avocado and Herb Salad

Prep Time 10 minutes

Ingredients

- Ripe firm avocados 2-3

- Lemon 1

- Green onions 3 thinly sliced

- Capers 2 tbsp

- Jalapeño pepper minced 1

- Fresh cilantro rough chopped and stems removed

- Fresh parsley rough chopped and stems removed the dressing

- Extra virgin olive oil 1/4 cup

- Orange blossom vinegar 3 tbsp

- Clove garlic minced 1

- Salt and black pepper

Instructions

1. Cut the avocado b/w thin slices & scatter it with the juice of a lemon .

2. Place them, including the capers, green onions, spices, & jalapeño, to a big shallow serving dish.

3. Stir together the dressing & drizzle it over the salad. Serve immediately with a fresh/new crushed coarse black pepper.

34. Fresh herb salad

Prep time 5 mins

Ingredients

- Baby arugula 2 oz. (2 cups)
- Fresh flat-leaf parsley leaves 1 cup
- Fresh mint leaves 1/2 cup
- Sliced fresh chives 2 Tbs.
- Fresh lemon juice 2 tsp
- Extra-virgin olive oil 2 tsp.
- Kosher salt and black pepper freshly ground

Preparation

- Toss together all the parsley, chives, arugula & mint in a med bowl.

- Mix together the juice of lemon & oil in a bowl & sprinkle with pepper & salt.

- Place over salad with the dressing. Toss to cover, then Serve right away.

35. Soft Herb Salad

Prep time 1 hour

Ingredients

For the loosely packed greens:

- Cilantro leaves 2 c

- Parsley leaves flat-leaf 1 c

- Small dill sprigs 1 c

- Basil/mint leaves 1 c

- Arugula leaves 1 c

- Purslane, Mache or lettuce leaves 2 c

For the dressing:

- Unsalted butter 4 tablespoons
- Sliced almonds 1 c
- Salt and black pepper coarsely ground
- Red chile flakes ¼ tsp or crushed pink peppercorns 1/2 tsp (optional)
- Lemon juice 3 tbsp
- Olive oil 2 tbsp

Preparation

1. Clean the herbs & greens up to a day before having to serve fill a clean sink/big bowl with plenty of cool water. Immerse the leaves, swing around to release some soil, and lift out nicely. Dry in a spinner of salads or spread on dry kitchen towels. (Cool the dry leaves in plastic bags or bins if you work ahead. Put a paper towel to every bag to retain excess water.)

2. Heat the butter till it sizzles in the pan. Put almonds. Sauté at low temperature, till the butter becomes

browned as well as the almonds become golden. Drop the almonds & drain with butter on paper towels. (Butter may be stored for 1 day. Before salad assembly, melt & cool again.

3. Put the greens in the wide bowl when they are ready to eat. Combine the salt, pepper, almonds, chili flakes, sugar, juice of lemon, & olive oil. Gently toss & sprinkle to taste. Serve right away.

36. All-natural tamarind paste

Prep time 1 hour

Ingredients:

- Natural tamarind 250 gr

- Springwater 3 cups

Instructions:

1. Get the tamarind clean. Search for any skin, unwanted particle, or any seed & remove them. Heat two glass of water, meanwhile.

2. For around 45-60 mins, soak your tamarind in two glass of hot water.

3. Till the tamarind is tender, mix this till really smooth in such a high-speed mixer. Pass your resulting combination through a fine-mesh strainer. Throw away any seeds, debris, or stones. Simmer the resultant pulp over a med flame for around five min.

4. Safe it in airtight containers when the paste is fully cooled.

37. Fantastic quinoa bread (Dr. Sebi)

Prep time 1 hr 30 min

For gluten intolerance/gluten sensitivity

Ingredients:

- Whole uncooked quinoa seed 300 g (1 3/4 cups)
- Water 1/2 cup
- Grapeseed oil 60 ml (¼ cup)
- Sea salt 1/2 teaspoon

- Key lime 1/2, juiced

Instructions:

1. Soak the quinoa in cool water in the refrigerator overnight. Oven preheated to 320 F/160 C.

2. Drain your quinoa & then rinse into a sieve very good. Be sure all the water is extracted from the sieve absolutely. Put the quinoa in a grinder mixer. Put 1/2 cup water, sea salt, grape seed oil, & lime juice.

3. For three minutes, blend in a grinder mixer. Batter stability with few full quinoas by now remaining in the mix could resemble the bread mix.

4. Cook for 1 1/2 hr till hard to touch & comes back when finger pressed.

5. Take it off the oven & chill in the pan for thirty min. After this, extract from the jar & chill on a rack fully. In the middle, the bread must be mildly moist & crisp on the outside.

6. Cool fully before serving. Now enjoy.

38. Tea Recipe Five Flavored Autumn

Prep time 35 mins

It soothes the nervous system, provides deep nourishment, and broadly supports the immune system.

Ingredients

- Dried astragalus 15 g
- Dried oat straw 10 g
- Dried rose hips de-seeded 10
- Dried dandelion root Roasted 10 g
- Dried cinnamon chips 3 g or cinnamon stick 1 broken into pieces
- Water 4 cups
- Apple juice 1 cup

Instructions

1. Put a med saucepan with the herbs & water. Boil it, now lower the heat & boil, protected, for thirty min. Switch

the heat off & put the juice of apple. Let sit for five min. Strain. Drink it warm/cool as you want.

39. Veggie fajitas tacos

Prep time 15 mins

Ingredients:

- Portobello mushrooms 2-3 large

- Bell peppers 2

- Onion 1

- 1/2 key lime juice of

- Corn-free tortillas 6 (look for approved grains tortillas, like Kamut flour tortillas)

- Avocado

- Approved seasonings (habanero, onion powder, cayenne pepper)

Instructions:

1. Remove the mushroom stems, spoon out the gills if necessary, & clean the tops. Split into pieces around 1/3 inch wide. Cut the bell peppers & onions thinly. On med heat in a wide skillet, put one Tbsp Grape seed oil, peppers & onions. Cook for around two min. Add toppings & mushrooms. Mix from time to time, cook for 7 to 8 mins or till softened.

2. Spoon a fajita combination into the middle of the tortillas & warm tortillas. Put avocado & key lime juice then serve.

40. Psyllium Apple & Lemon Balm Tea

Prep time: 5mins

The psyllium husk retains moisture through the digestive system and develops a gel-like material, which facilitates bowel movements. Also, It helps decrease the absorption of fat from the intestine. If you do not have the lemon balm tea, you should use cold water, since this tea form has been found to have slight sedative results. It can help to control the blood sugar by using pure cinnamon, which will, in turn, boost insulin sensitivity & minimize the sugar conversion into stored fat.

Ingredients:

- Apple 1

- Lemon balm tea 1 cup, cooled

- Psyllium husk powder 2 tsp

- True cinnamon ¼ tsp

Instructions:

1. Combine all the ingredients completely & drink.

41. Aloe Vera Cherry Juice

Prep time: 5mins

For increasing, melatonin levels in people. This hormone regulates the sleeping cycle and enhances sleep.

Ingredients:

- Coldwater 1 cup

- Aloe vera juice 1 oz

- Tart cherry juice 2-4 oz

Instructions:

1. Mix together all the ingredients till smooth in a well-speed grinder. Enjoy it.

42. Sugar detox smoothie

Prep time: 5mins

Sipping on a greens drink can help reduce sugar cravings, especially if you have it on an empty stomach.

Ingredients:

- Avocado 1/2
- Soft-jelly coconut milk homemade 1 cup
- Approved greens 1 handful, like callaloo, dandelion greens, or watercress
- Key lime squeeze 1
- Bromide Plus Powder (Dr. Sebi) 1 teaspoon

Instructions:

1. In a high-speed processor, mix all the ingredients & enjoy it.

43. Heart-healthy smoothie

Prep time: 5mins

Besides the heart-healthy fats from the nuts, this apple smoothie features the cholesterol-lowering soluble fiber from the apples and walnut milk and antioxidants from the blueberries.

Ingredients:

- Braeburn apple 1, or another kind of organic apple
- Brazil nuts 1/4 cup
- Homemade walnut milk 1 cup
- Blueberries 1 cup
- Approved greens 1 cup (dandelion greens, watercress, turnip greens, etc.)
- Date sugar/agave syrup 1/2 tablespoon

Instructions:

1. Blend all the ingredients together in a high-speed blender and enjoy.

44. Immunity-boosting soup

Prep time: 10 mins

Comfort in a bowl. Enjoy this alkaline-electric, nutrient-packed bowl of immunity-boosting soup.

Ingredients:

- Onion 1/2

- Bell pepper 1

- Mushrooms 1 cup (any kind, except shiitake)

- Grapeseed oil 1 tablespoon

- Approved flour noodles 1 pack (spelt, wild rice, amaranth, etc.)

- Key lime 1

- Zucchini 1

- Cherry tomatoes 1 cup

- Water cups 4

- Herbs (Approved)

- Cayenne pepper and Sea salt

Instructions:

1. As per the package directions, cook the noodles.

2. Mince the onion into tiny cubes. Warm the grapeseed oil in a wide saucepan & sauté onion till it is translucent.

3. Chop little bits of mushrooms, cherry tomatoes & bell pepper. Sauté in a pan, too. Chop the Courgette & put it the pan.

4. Add the sea salt, spices, pepper & water. Carry it over med heat to a simmer. Reduce the heat until the boiling point is hit. Place the noodles that have been cooked. Let it boil for ten more mins.

5. Adjust toppings. Serve with key juice of lime & also with more herbs.

45. Nori-burritos

Prep time: 10 mins

These alkaline-electric seaweed rolls are packed with alkaline-electric, portable nutrition. We are sure you'll enjoy this fresh wraps.

Ingredients:

- Ripe avocado 1
- Cucumber (seeded) 450 gr
- Ripe mango 1/2
- Nori seaweed 4 sheets
- Zucchini 1, small
- Amaranth/dandelion greens (handful)
- sprouted hemp seeds (handful)
- Tahini 1 tbs
- Sesame seeds

Instructions:

1. Put the Nori sheet on a chopping board.

2. Assemble all of the ingredients on the nori sheet, leaving the exposed nori to the right with an inch broad margin.

3. Fold the nori sheet from the edge nearest to you with the hands, folding it up & on the fillings. Season with sesame seeds & cut into thick pieces.

46. Lemon-Ginger and Chamomile Tea

Prep time: 5mins

- Chamomile tea 6 oz
- Cucumber with skin 5 to 10 slices
- Freshly grated ginger 1 tbsp
- Lemon 1 juiced
- (optional) Himalayan salt pinch

Instructions:

1. Mix all these ingredients to have an enjoyable pre-bedtime drink.

47. Iron power smoothie

Prep time: 5mins

Boost the iron levels in your blood with this delicious apple smoothie. The "Iron Power" Smoothie will help you fight iron deficiency.

Ingredients:

- Red apple large 1/2

- Currants/raisins 1 tbsp.

- Fig 1

- Cooked quinoa 1/2 cup

- Hemp seed milk homemade 1 cup

- Handfuls amaranth greens 2

- Date sugar 1 tbsp.

- Bromide + powder 1 tsp.

Instructions:

1. Mix everything till smooth in a high-powerful processor & enjoy.

48. Dr. Sebi's "stomach soother" smoothie

Prep time: 5mins

For Cramping, Indigestion, Bloating, Pain. For digestive problems and stomach ache woes with the delicious Dr. Sebi's Stomach Soother Smoothie.

Ingredients:

- Burro banana 1
- Prepared 1/2 cup stomach relief herbal tea (dr. Sebi's)
- Ginger tea 1/2 cup
- Agave syrup 1 tbsp.

Instructions:

1. As commanded, make the tea allow it to cool. Mix with the rest of the ingredients & enjoy.

49. Dr. Sebi's "veggie-ful" smoothie

Prep time: 5mins

Ingredients:

- Pear 1, cored & seeded

- Avocado 1/4

- Seeded cucumber 1/2, peeled

- Handful watercress 1

- Romaine lettuce 1 handful

- Springwater 1/2 cup

- (optional) Date sugar

Instructions:

1. In a high-powerful processor, mix together all the ingredients till smooth. Enjoy.

50. Detox watercress citrus salad

Prep time: 10 mins

The Watercress Citrus Salad is highly nutritious, full of antioxidants and minerals, and absolutely refreshing and delicious.

Ingredients:

- Ripe Avocado 1

- Watercress 4 cups

- Seville orange 1, zested, sliced& peeled

- red onion very thin slices 2

- agave syrup 2 tsp.

- Key lime juice 2 tbsp.

- Olive oil 2 tbsp.

- Salt 1/8 tsp.

- optional Cayenne pepper

Instructions:

1. Put avocado, watercress, oranges & onion on a plate or two. In a shallow bowl, combine the olive oil, key lime juice, salt, cayenne pepper & agave syrup together. Once ready to eat, spoon the dressing on the salad.

51. Cucumber basil gazpacho

Prep time: 15 mins

The Cucumber Basil Gazpacho is a creamy-tasting chilled soup, a natural for serving as an appetizer in small glasses or as a light lunch or supper on hot summer days.

Ingredients:

- Ripe avocado perfectly 1

- Seeded cucumber 1: skin left; seeds removed

- Handfuls fresh basil 2 small

- Water 2 cups

- Sea salt 1 1/4 teaspoon

- 1 key lime juice

Instructions:

1. To cook this cold soup called "gazpacho." Put all the ingredients in the fridge till cold. Put in a blender & purée the cooled ingredients until smooth, leaving several green specks to stay while. Place the soup back in the refrigerator and cool before ready for serving. Sprinkle with leaves of basil & cucumber circles that are thinly cut.

52. Dandelion strawberry salad

Prep time: 10 mins

Dandelion greens are used in traditional medicine to treat many ailments. Recent studies have shown that dandelion kills certain bacteria and other microbes, and it even has anti-cancer properties. Try them in a salad that mixes sweet and savory flavors with heavenly results.

Ingredients:

- Grapeseed oil 2 tbsp.

- Sliced medium red onion 1

- Strawberries ripe sliced 10

- Key lime juice 2 tbsp.

- Dandelion greens 4 cups

- Sea salt

Instructions:

1. In a 12-inch nonstick frying pan, melt grape seed oil over low pressure. Along with a strong pinch of sea salt,

apply sliced onions. Cook until the onions are smooth, slightly orange, and reduced to about 1/3 of the raw amount, stirring regularly.

2. In a shallow bowl, toss 1 tsp of key juice of a lime with the raspberry slices. Clean the dandelion greens &, if you prefer, break them into bite-sized bits. Add the rest key juice of a lime to a skillet once the onions are almost cooked & continue frying till the onions are thickened, a min /two to coat. Take off the heat from the onions. Mix the onions, raspberries & greens with all of their juices in a salad dish. Season with sea salt.

53. Wakame salad

Prep time: 10 mins

Sea vegetables are loaded with antioxidants, fiber, and iodine. This Wakame salad is a tasty – and definitely not boring – way to eat your greens.

Ingredients:

- Wakame stems 2 cups
- Onion powder 1 teaspoon

- Ginger 1 teaspoon

- Red bell pepper 1 tablespoon

- Sesame seeds 1 tablespoon

- Key lime juice 1 tablespoon

- Agave syrup 1 tablespoon

- Sesame oil 1 tablespoon

Instructions:

1. Soak the wakame stems and drain for 5 to 10 mins.

2. Mix the sesame seed, key lime juice, agave syrup, powder of onion & ginger in a food processor. Mix completely. Put the wakame & bell pepper in a dish to eat. On top, place dressing. Season with sesame seeds

54. Super hydrating smoothie

Prep time: 5mins

Dr. Sebi's Super Hydrating Smoothie contains natural electrolytes from the soft-jelly coconut water and tons of minerals from the watermelon and strawberries. This is an excellent, refreshing option to keep you hydrated during hot summer months.

Ingredients:

- Strawberries 1 cup
- watermelon chunks 1 cup
- date sugar 1 tbsp.
- soft jelly coconut water 1 cup

Instructions:

1. Mix together all the ingredients.

Conclusion

An herb is a plant or product component for its smell, taste, or medicinal characteristics. One form of dietary supplement is herbal medications. They are marketed as capsules, tablets, powders, extracts, teas, and new or dry plants. Herbal drugs are used by people to attempt to preserve or enhance their wellbeing. Natural herbs play a huge part in healing our bodies

Cultures and countries have relied on conventional herbal medicine for centuries to fulfill their healthcare needs. The global market for herbal medicines is on the rise, amid the modern age's medical and technical advances. In reality, this industry is expected to gross about 60 billion dollars annually. Many natural remedies can be more efficient and convenient than traditional medications, and since they fit with their personal wellbeing ideologies, many people choose to use them.

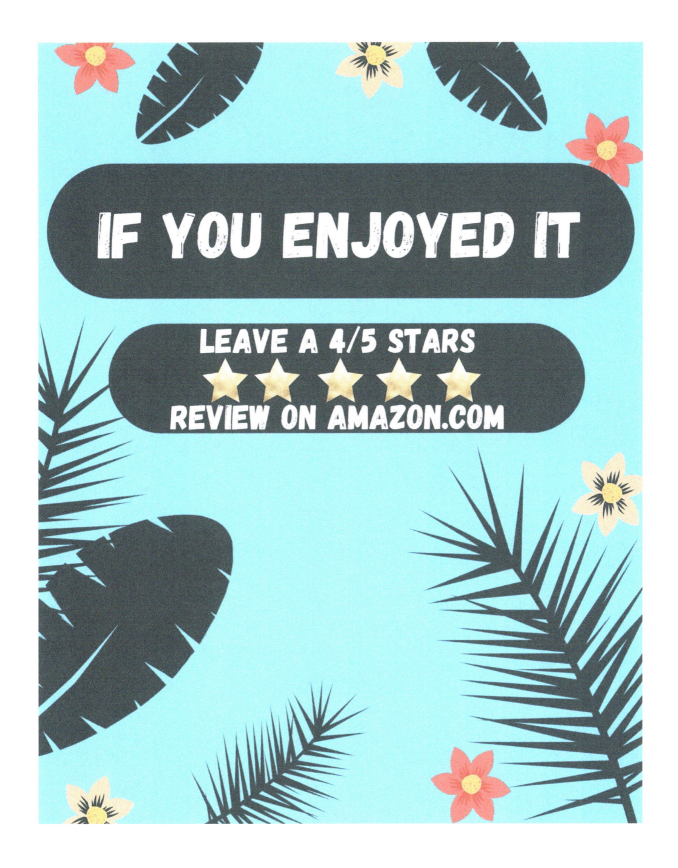